I0423609

Also by Dr. Stenbeck

Available from the usual on-line source

Books

Healing Yourself -- The Holistic Approach
  [An introduction to Holistic Self-healing.]

Heal Yourself Right Now!
  *[The Seven Priority Organ Levels for
  effective Nutritional/Holistic Treatment of
  all organs.]*

The 22 Unique Body Types
  (for Health and Weight Loss)

Q & A to Identify Your Body Type (Booklet)
  [Individual Type booklets are also available

Booklets
(Step-by-step instructions on healing yourself)

  #1 Start Healing with Positive Thinking
  #2 Mastering Positive Feelings for Health!
  #3 Spiritual Balance and Your Healing

The Marasmic Body Type

Representing one of the 22 Body Types first described by Victor Rocine around 1900

The President Obama, Princess Diana Celebrity Body Type

Copyright © 2017

by Dr. Lloyd Stenbeck

All rights reserved.

Except as permitted by the Copyright Act of 1976, no part of this publication may be used or reproduced, distributed, or transmitted in any form or by any means, electronic, recording, photocopy, mechanical, including or stored in a database, or any information storage and retrieval system without the prior written permission of the author.

First Edition: 2017

For Kaye,
there at the beginning with Doc Severn,
and for Liberty,
continuing the holistic healing journey…

Disclaimer

The information in this book is for educational purposes only and is not a substitute for medication, diets, or other medical care. The diets do not treat diseases or medical conditions, and are an adjunct to your orthodox health care.

The author and publisher accept no responsibility for any misuse of the information within. If you have any physical problem, food allergy, emotional disorder, or disease, common sense dictates that you consult with a physician before changing your diet, taking nutritional supplements, or following the advice given here.

———

About the Author

Educated in New Zealand and in the U.S.A., Dr. Stenbeck attained B.Sc. (NZ), M.S., and D.C. degrees. His holistic healing methods have been profiled in magazines (Esquire, McLean's, Playgirl, the Atlanta Constitution), and on TV in the USA and in Canada. He was the main contributor to the Warner Book, _The Eye/Body Connection_ by Jessica Maxwell that focused on the holistic healing relationships between the iris structure and organ genetics.

In the 1970-80's he was elected Fellow, Royal Society of Health, London; Fellow, American Association of Chemists; Member, American Association of Clinical Chemists; and Affiliate, Royal Society of Medicine, London. He studied naturopathy and Body Types with Dr. Bernard Jensen and Dr. Clifford Severn, and has practiced in medical partnerships where patients received the joint benefits of medical and holistic healing.

He is a member of Self-Realization Fellowship. To receive advice on any health issue from a holistic viewpoint, or to receive help with your body type, see his web site: *DrStenbeck.net*

———

Contents

* * *

The Marasmic Body Type and Food Guide   1

* * *

The 22 Body Types: Celebrity Examples

This Booklet contains the Marasmic type. See <u>The 22 Unique Body Types</u> for all type descriptions.]

Thin Types

Atrophic	*Woody Allen / Audrey Hepburn* *Stan Laurel / Calista Flockheart*
Exesthesic	*Cher / Sarah Jessica Parker* *(Female type only)*
Marasmic	*President Obama / Princess Diana* *James Stewart / Kate Blanchard*
Neurogenic	*J.K. Simmons / Joan Rivers* *Jon Cryer / Marin Hinle*
Pathoferic	*(No celebrity males)* *Blythe Danner / Gwyneth Paltrow*
Sillevitic	*David Bowie / Shirley MacLaine* *Rod Stewart / Carol Channing*

Muscle Types

Calciferic	*Michael Jordan / Angelica Huston*
	Abraham Lincoln / Grace Jones
Carbogenic	*George Clooney / Lady Gaga*
	Pres. G. Bush, Jr. / Meg Ryan
Desmogenic	*Marlon Brando / Loni Anderson*
	Daniel Craig / Tina Turner
Eldic	*Ross Perot / Hillary Clinton*
	Peter Falk / Sigourney Weaver
Myogenic	*Pres. Bill Clinton / Sharon Stone*
	Pres. John Kennedy / Julia Roberts
Nervimotive	*Frank Sinatra / Elizabeth Taylor*
	Mark Wahlberg / Natalie Wood
Nitropheric	*Ben Affleck / Ava Gardner*
	Kirk Douglas / Kate Winslet
Pallinomic	*Pres. Donald Trump /*
	Attorney General Janet Reno
	Bill O'Reilly (Fox) / Jane Russell

Fat Types

Barotic   *Robin Williams / 'Mrs. Doubtfire'*
      Elton John / William Conrad

Carboferic *Bill Murray / Roseanne*
      Billy Gardell / Melissa McCarthy

Hydripheric *John Goodman / Shelly Winters*
      Wayne Knight / Jennifer Holliday

Isogenic   *Einstein / Oprah Winfrey*
      Phillip S. Hoffman / Queen Victoria

Lipopheric *Rush Limbaugh / Rosie O'Donnell*
      Chris Christie / Camryn Manheim

Oxypheric *Winston Churchill / Orsen Welles*
      Ella Fitzgerald / Gerry Spence

Pargenic   *Burt Reynolds / Katey Segal*
      Ron Perlman / Kirstey Alley

Succinct Quote on Human Types

From Victor Rocine, who first described discrete body types around 1900.

"A type is an order of people that differentiates and distinguishes itself by a general and similar form, brain-formation, chemistry, structure, build, immunity, tendencies, predisposition, resemblance, skin-pigment, and type characteristics based on observation and analogy.

"Or, in other words, people of a given type are similar physically and like-minded as if they were brothers and sisters—that is what type means.

"Everything in nature is made according to plan. Man only discovers that plan and gives it a name. The zoologist has not made the animals—he has only described the plan adopted by the wonderful Creator, and named the classes, sub-classes, etc.

"How important type research will be to humanity, time alone will make known."

———

Prologue

The esteemed scientist J. J. Berzelius, discoverer of several chemical elements, inspired Victor Rocine to research body types and to investigate the correlation between types and their diseases. Around 1890-1910, Rocine privately published his original findings on the mineral basis of different body types, and this present book exists because of his brilliant insights.

For many years, I studied with Dr. Clifford Severn who had been a personal student of Victor Rocine on body types, naturopathy, herbology, iris analysis, diet, and nutritional healing methods. He had a successful career as a lecturer and healer, and was one of those rare athletes with complete muscle control over his body. I saw him under a spotlight at 85 years of age, contracting and rippling every individual muscle in his perfectly developed body. Field-Marshal Jan Smuts, the WWII South African Prime Minister, devoted a full chapter of his autobiography to how Severn's healing methods had saved his life. In the 1950's, *Life* magazine did a four-page spread on Severn and his family. Fame he had.

Another Rocine student I studied with, Dr. Bernard Jensen wrote of Rocine's body type research and nutritional methods in his privately published book *The Chemistry of Man*.

This book is deeply rooted in Rocine's original work, and with that of Herbert Shelton, M.D., Ph.D. (at Harvard University in the 1930's). I integrated their research with newer dietary and nervous system data along with celebrity examples of each type, hopefully, making this material easier to digest and more entertaining for the reader.

Gayelord Hauser, another Rocine student I knew, was a celebrated health book author. He wrote a popular book on Rocine's types in the 1940's, *Types and Temperaments;* reputedly, he also introduced yogurt to the western world.

This book exists because of Rocine's creative brilliance and original discoveries in natural healing.

▶ *Rocine: "The soul creates the body type."*

Rocine taught that the soul chooses a body type and brain to live in, thus presenting different experiences and life lessons to master. Why were *you* born the way you are?

That is something to think about, especially if it is true! What would your soul purpose be to live in a particular body type. I provide some thoughts on this issue in each type description and try to assess from my experience with your type the particular lessons of life presented therein.

Rocine was as brilliant in his way as an Abraham Lincoln, Michael Jordan, Michael Phelps, Tony Robbins, or a Daniel Day Lewis—all *calciferic* types—rare, leaders, innovative, brilliant, and highly intelligent in their different fields of endeavor.

Celebrity examples exist for most types, not a duplicate of you, but someone who has your essence in their body-mind individuality. Knowing your type allows you to become a better you!

The celebrity examples provide further help in identifying your body type.

▶ *Rocine's classic findings are the backbone of this book. Integrated with Sheldon's research and with other dietary and food issues including mental, emotional, and spiritual attributes,*

Many people take nutritional supplements and try different diets without a doctor's advice. If this is your choice, use common sense, listen to body responses, and discontinue any allergic reactions to foods or nutritional substances.

———

The Marasmic
Body Type

"You may also have a physical or psychological feature not representative of your type such as height, weight, appearance, talent, weakness, strength, etc., due to biochemical errors, environmental influences, racial or cultural differences, and congenital or genetic issues. Nevertheless, the type identification of the average person is usually clear."

—Victor Rocine

Marasmic Type
Celebrity Examples

If you think this is your type, be sure to look at **on-line photographs** *of these examples. Look for general similarities to yourself. Note that sub-types cause the differences in appearance between members of the same type.*

———

ROYALTY

Princess Diana

POLITICS

President George H. W. Bush, Sr.
Senator Alan Cranston
Presidential Candidate Bernie Sanders

ACTING (Many actors, many Oscars!)

Clint Eastwood	Alan Alda
Peter O'Toole	Leonard Nimoy
Bruce Dern	Laurence Harvey
Frank Langella	Ben Cross
Jeff Goldblum	Michael Redgrave
Dennis Weaver	Gary Cooper
Richard Chamberlain	Mel Ferrer
Danny Kaye	Timothy Hutton
Donald Sutherland	Dick Van Dyke

James Stewart   Henry Fonda
Jeremy Irons   Bela Lugosi
Max Von Sydow   Scott Glenn
Peter Coyote   Raymond Massey
Peter Cushing   Boris Karloff
Jason Robards   Rex Harrison
Harry Anderson   Robert Ryan

Lucille Ball   Lynn Redgrave
Laura Dern   Vanessa Redgrave
Jane Lynch   Allison Janney

TV

Charlie Rose   Tom Snyder

SPORTS *(may have great athletic potential)*

Mickey Mantle   Joe DiMaggio
Kevin Johnson   Darryl Strawberry
Bill Walton   John Isner
Kareem Abdul Jabbar

MUSIC

Barry Manilow   Harry Connick Jr.

ARTS/OTHER

Arthur Miller   Ted Turner
Jim Henson   Charles Keating
Howard Hughes

Quite a list! I knew two of the above celebrities, numerous others in everyday life, and in my family, which contributed to my understanding of the type.]

You already know something about this type from their public persona and appearance, whether from seeing them yourself or from the celebrity examples. Blend such insights with the type descriptions and the types of your family and friends to discern their presence in your midst!

Read the types, and if still confusedyou may choose to use the personal request for type identification from my web site: *DrStenbeck.net*

———

Marasmic Type Questionnaire

These questions describe the generic type, and not specifically you! If any question ever applied to you, then choose the True answer!

For Question 1 only:

A = True	*B = Maybe*	*C = Untrue*
15 points	*7 points*	*1 point*

1. Physically identify with celebrity example____

Then...

A = True	*B = Maybe*	*C = Untrue*
5 points	*3 points*	*1 point*

---

2. Height is usually close to:
   Males: 6'0-6'11   Females: 5'10-6'6   ____
3. Usual weight (pounds) is close to:
   Males: 150-230 Females: 140-185   ____
4. Slender or gaunt body, weight easily
   controlled until older (may gain
   30-40 pounds with a fat sub-type)   ____
5. Moderate strength, able to body-build ____
6. Robust, strong love-making capacity
   and sexual drive (especially males)   ____
7. Able to manage people   ____
8. Hair is fine and dry; some have a
   thinning tendency; sparse beard   ____
9. Are assertive and aggressive if needed ____

10. Teeth usually large and strong _____
11. Have strong willpower; can take action in any situation _____
12. A few are star athletes (some *neurogenics* and *sillevitics*) _____
13. Marked cheekbones, sunken cheeks _____
14. Smaller lower jaw and chin _____
15. May have a sunken, bony chest; narrow from front to back; slight chest hair growth _____
16. Skin typically dry with fine wrinkles _____
17. Often sarcastic if provoked _____
18. Excellent coordination _____
19. Have teaching talents _____
20. Voice authoritative, impressive _____
21. Forehead tends to retreat backwards _____
22. Many fine aging lines in the face _____
23. May worry a lot about health _____
24. Reserved, private, and withdrawn _____
25. Weight gain is slow (and easily lost) _____
26. Use friendly persuasion with others _____
27. Stoical and dogmatic _____
28. Some may be inconsiderate _____
29. Most are honorable and ethical _____
30. Some are cynical and pessimistic _____
31. Waistline well controlled early in life _____
32. High self-confidence and self-image _____
33. Always thin, tall, lean; some medium-height, but never short _____
34. Females attractive, rarely beautiful; males ruggedly handsome _____
35. Quick learners, talented _____

36. Gentle and exclusive qualities _____
37. Head is rectangular shape, longer
      from front to back _____
38. Face long, pleasant looking; prom-
      inent cheekbones, sunken cheeks _____
39. Joints weak, easily injured; bones long,
      stronger than most thin types _____
40. Good leadership abilities _____
41. Deformed or weak chest structure is
      common; small bust _____
42. Many are original and creative _____
43. Calm, cool, reserved, and withdrawn _____
44. Have a tough demeanor _____
45. Stubborn tendency _____
46. May be controlling in relationships _____
47. Express opinions honestly _____
48. Confident in social situations _____
49. Unconfident in romantic situations _____
50. Cultured and sensitive _____
51. Intelligent and ambitious _____
52. String need to feel loved _____
53. Many are courageous and heroic _____
54. Strong leadership ability _____
55. Some have monogamy problems _____
56. Talented in mental and creative work,
      arts, sales, teaching _____
57. May be shy and awkward, especially _____
58. Dislike hard physical labor _____
59. Most have strong calcium metabolism,
      teeth, and gums—if healthy _____

Scoring

For question #1:
A response: give 15 points   =_____
B response: give 7 points   =_____
C response: give 1 ,points   =_____

For questions #2—59:
A response: give 5 points   =_____
B response: give 3 points   =_____
C response: give 1 point   =_____

Total of the above points   =_____

Interpretation
145—275: PROBABLY Marasmic type
80—144: POSSIBLY Marasmic type
<80: NOT Marasmic type

The Marasmic Type

Rocine: "'Marasmic' means 'wasted and lean'—only the atrophic type is more lean-looking. You absorb and utilize from your diet excessive amounts of <u>chloride and calcium</u> compared to other types making you lean and bony." [And... I would add, intelligent.]

———

Physically you are always tall and slender, but after age 40 you may gain about 10 to 30 pounds on a high calorie diet. You are the strongest Thin type with most tall and slender professional basketball, baseball, and tennis players being of your type (for example, Kareem Abdul Jabbar, Joe DiMaggio, and John Isner). Such athletes have a superior blend of body-mind coordination with moderate strength (whereas the *atrophic* type is rarely athletic).

If female, you are attractive but rarely beautiful, Princess Diana being an obvious exception. The males are ruggedly handsome as in Gary Cooper and James Stewart. You are a quick learner, talented, brilliant, and original in your thinking, and are found at all levels of society. You achieve your goals.

Chloride, a thinning element, helps take fat out of your tissues, and is excessively absorbed and utilized by the *marasmic, atrophic and medeic* types. Calcium makes you bony, moderately strong, and tall like President G. Bush, Sr. *Marasmics* are mental, practical, creative, intelligent, and able to take care of business and to get things done. Some of you may be inconsiderate, but mostly you are gentle and reserved.

▶ *You always need to avoid salt (sodium chloride) and salty foods, and should eat high calorie foods when younger. Your metabolism is wired to slenderness although you may gain extra pounds in later years.*

―――

Physical Similarity to Other Types

You are often confused with the much leaner *atrophic* type, or the very rare *calciferic* type.

The *atrophic* type (Tony Perkins, Audrey Hepburn) is thin or lean, and physically weak.

The *calciferic* type (James Coburn, Grace Jones) is always tall, bony, lean, strong, highly intelligent, balding, and unmistakable.

The *nitropheric* type (Gregory Peck, Jessica Lang) may be quite lean and tall when young.

The taller *neurogenic* male (J.K. Simmons) is lean and balding.

The taller *sillevitic* type (David Bowie) is lean, strong, and attractive or handsome.

———

Average Height and Weight

| Males: | 6'0-6'11 | 150-230 | pounds |
| Females: | 5'10-6'6 | 140-175 pounds | |

———

Marasmic Type Description

The type description represents how you appear in everyday society. You may have a sub-type that alters parts of this description.

You may be lean from excessive chloride intake, but less-so than the *atrophic* (the thinnest of all types). You may rarely have a fat or muscle sub-type thereby maintaining a more medium-sized body.

Head — Your head is rectangular, typically narrow, and long from the front to back, the forehead usually retreats backwards.

Hair — You have dry thin hair, usually brown; balding is rare.

Eyes — Mostly sunken and brown eyes, some blue.

Ears — You usually have average-sized ears, sometimes larger due to an *eldic* sub-type.

Nose — A long and thin nose with pinched nostrils is typical.

Face — You have a long pleasant face, without the irregular features seen in *atrophic* males; you usually have prominent cheekbones, sunken cheeks, and a receding chin.

Mouth, Lips and Voice — An average-sized mouth is common. Your voice is usually quiet, understated, and authoritative.

Teeth — Active calcium metabolism provides moderate strength of teeth and gums (with effective childhood calcium absorption).

Skin — You typically have dry skin with fine wrinkles.

Neck — A long thin and scrawny neck is common.

Muscles — You have moderate muscle strength. You may have a good ability in low-impact sports like tennis, baseball, basketball, etc., with some superstars!

▶ *You have good brain-muscle coordination as seen in a great athlete like Mickey Mantle; you are the strongest of the thin types, but weak compared to the muscle and fat types. A few of you become long distance runners, Olympians, and pro-athletes with great coordination and balance.*

Back and Shoulders — Your broad back and shoulders slant down to a narrow waist.

Hips and Abdomen — A flat abdomen is the rule; the hips are thin and narrow.

Chest — You have a flat, bony and thin chest; the males have sparse hair growth, and some have deformed rib-cages; a small or absent bust is usual.

Arms and Legs — Your extremities are strong, long and lean.

Joints — The joints are easily injured, and your long, durable, and flexible bones are strong compared to the *atrophic.*

———

Marasmic Personality Traits

If you are this type many, but not all, of the following characteristics are present—you may have overcome or moderated the negatives, but recognize that once you had several of them.

Positive Qualities

You may show any of the following traits:

- Assertive, some quite aggressive
- Good sense of humor, witty, comical
- Great methodical trustworthy workers
- Have high self-confidence and self-image
- Confident, friendly, ethical, and dependable
- Are humane, intelligent, leaders, and honest
- High courage, integrity, and strong willpower
- Calm, withdrawn, stoical, heroic, and honorable

Potential Challenges

You may have evolved from, or not experienced these general faults, so do not dwell on them:

- Anxiety, fear around intimacy
- Some have cravings or addictions

- Tend to be shy, reserved, and controlling
- Some may be withdrawn, cynical, pessimistic
- Stubborn, may unknowingly offend people with frank opinions
- Males may have doubts around approaching the opposite sex, and suffer from low self-esteem, worth, and acceptance
- Appear friendly, kind, loving, some have a tough demeanor (many of the celebrity examples had roles needing toughness and arrogance)

► *If you relate to any of these challenges, doing something to overcome them serves your evolution.*

———

Marasmic Stress Management

You have strong mental stress prevention giving you a good ability
stress into your sto
immune system. Emotional stress prevention is vulnerable, and any of the above challenges may need reprogramming help. *If needing help managing these stresses, see ;*

———

Love

Rocine: "You are often attracted to the *calciferic, carbogenic, desmogenic, eldic, nervimotive, pathoferic, nitropheric, and pargenic* types, and have a strong sexual drive and love-making ability." (The *atrophic* has a strong drive with less endurance.)

———

Talents and Vocations

Abilities - *Artistic, healing, sales*

You are cultured, sensitive, studious, intelligent, ambitious, and born for thinking and creative work. You are widely found in management positions, and often excel in leadership and in the military (unlike the *atrophic*).

I have known you as bookkeepers, homemakers, authors, electricians, monastics, teachers, doctors, inventors, handymen, musicians, plumbers, carpenters, engineers, accountants, investors, electrical engineers, computer specialists, office managers, film producers and directors, and creative heads of industry. Jobs requiring mind-hand skills attract you like carpentry, plumbing, etc. You swing a hammer with the best of them!

The type information cannot predict what or who you will become, but you are capable of bringing a creative excellence or brilliance to whatever you do in life.

Inabilities - *Hard physical labor, law*

Heavy labor is not your forte. You respond to your feelings, readily speak your mind, and therefore cannot be a skilled attorney where you need to think on your feet.

———

Health Problems

When sick you commonly experience health problems or diseases in any of the following organs and tissues:

Spine, Bones and Joints — These tissues are moderately strong; osteoporosis is common requiring phosphorus foods.

Liver and Kidneys — These organs are weak, prone to toxicity, allergies, inefficiency, and water-weight problems.

Lungs — Collapsed lungs and bronchial diseases are common.

Sinuses — Are vulnerable to chronic infect-ions; allergies are frequent.

Chronic Infections — Females often experience recurrent infections.

Immune Organs — Are weak making you vulnerable to infection.

———

Marasmic Acid/Alkaline Factor

For your health and healing, the genetics of your autonomic nervous system predispose you to needing a specific ratio of food acidity to alkalinity. You are born with a slightly acid constitution, which means you need a slightly **alkaline-ash** food intake for acid/alkaline balance; about (Ash refers to the minerals left in your body after metabolizing foods.) Your nervous system genetics have *sympathetic* nervous system dominance. Construct this approximate ratio of food selections:

60% Fruits, salads, vegetables
40% Proteins, carbohydrates

[See Chapter 3 for details on this subject, along with the common symptoms found with people of different nervous system dominance.]

———

The Marasmic Spiritual Factor

Skip this paragraph if uninterested in a philosophical perspective on your body type!

▶ *Rocine: "The soul chooses the body type."*

If as souls, we choose the brain and body type to spend a lifetime in, it could be to learn certain spiritual lessons related to perfecting ourselves, and our humanity, in God's eyes. What lessons does the type bring you? Only you can really decide what those lessons are. You know your weaknesses, faults, and behaviors towards others. You know things about yourself that Victor Rocine could never get from his research subjects when he first wrote about types. So search your mind for the answers.

Each discrete type has challenges of life lessons, spiritual goals, etc., and some of yours may be:

Faith — You may maintain a strong faith, particularly if brought up in a religion. Consider that God may exist, and that you need to explore this possibility.

Arrogant or Aloof — You may feel superior to other people and thereby need humility lessons.

Fear of Intimacy — Excessive anxiety or self-doubt around the opposite sex is common to this type due to low self: esteem and worth.

Controlling — Some of you like to control situations and other people. Relinquish any need to control others and surrender control of your life to God.

Cold and Reserved — You may need to loosen up, smile and practice more friendliness with people. You may unknowingly offend people with your frank opinions and actions (especially males).

Impatience — Work at overcoming this negative trait: develop patience with those of inferior intellects! Overcome any egotism and negative judgments of others. Therapy helps!

Cravings, Addictions — Ask your friends and loved ones if you have a problem as you are often in denial about alcohol, drugs, or sex addictions (especially males). You may have an addictive tendency: if a careful social drinker and not using drugs, then no problem. Such vulnerability may only show with foods, sugar, etc., or it may be an unhealthy addiction.

▶ *If you relate to any of the above challenges, doing something to overcome them serves your evolution.*

_____

A Marasmic Story...

Freddie, 36, 175 pounds, 6'3, had primary complaints of apathy and fear. I found excessive chloride foods in his diet: milk, cheese (Brie, Roquefort, and Swiss), salt-water fish, processed foods (dill pickles, sauerkraut, meats, and frozen vegetables). In addition, his diet was high in red meats, poultry, and fish—opposite to his body type requirements! He needed a partial *vegetarian* diet to set the scene for his health restoration!

Over the next few weeks, Freddie corrected his *Food Guide* issues. His problems started resolving, and were soon under complete control.

_____

Marasmic Type
Mineral Food Needs

Apply this mineral data to the diet following the Thin type descriptions.

Excessive Foods:

- *Chlorine (salt, junk foods)*
- *Calcium*
- *Nitrogen (beef)*

Deficient Foods:

- *Carbon*
- *Phosphorus*
- *Sodium (unsalted, non-junk)*
- *Magnesium*
- *Nitrogen (non-beef, vegetable)*

These deficient nutrients are common deficiencies in your type, and predispose you to ill-health.
If ill, be sure to use these lists with your daily food intake. If not ill, eat from the food lists 3-4 days weekly for health maintenance.
All food lists are in descending order of concentration and value to you, choose servings of foods in the upper half of each list first! One serving is ½ cup.

Marasmic Excessive Foods -

Chlorine from salted junk foods and the salt shaker contributes to aging and to negative emotional states. Avoid it.

Calcium is excessively absorbed in your tissues, and is concentrated in your bones, joints, muscles, nerves, heart, teeth, and gums; calcium supplements rarely are needed. Phosphorus deficiency may interfere with your calcium metabolism.

Nitrogen from red meat, if eaten more than 1-2 times monthly, is excessive in your diet and contributes to your acidity and illness; if not vegetarian, eat poultry, fish and eggs 3-4 days weekly, with vegetarian proteins like legumes, seeds, nuts, and pasta on the other days.

———

Deficient Foods -

In illness or disease, it is important to correct these mineral deficiencies.

Carbon may be deficient in your tissues; it builds more flesh on your body. It is excessive in all fat people and is found in every cell of the body as the basis of life. If underweight, eat more of these foods.

Phosphorus, deficient in your tissues because of intense nervous system activity and brain exhaustion, helps balance your calcium metabolism. You think and worry about many things in your life.

Sodium as *unsalted* sodium foods is deficient in your type. Sodium is needed in all body types to help eliminate calcium deposition in joints, arteries, and soft tissues. In illness or disease, sodium excess from salted foods, along with a deficiency of *unsalted* sodium foods, are important factors in your healing.

Magnesium tends to be deficient in your type, and is particularly important for your heart and digestive function.

Nitrogen from vegetable sources is deficient (see above notes).

[See the Appendix for descriptions of mineral functions in the body.]

Minimize
Excessive Foods

Chlorine: *0-1 servings/week*

Milk, kelp, olives, lobster, Swiss chard, beet greens, celery
And: these chlorine, salted junk foods
Salt, all fast foods, packaged foods, canned and frozen foods, preserved meats (cured, smoked, canned), sauces (soy, barbecue, catsup, etc.), chips (potato, corn, etc.), dill pickles, sauerkraut, bouillon cubes, peanut butter, salted nuts, crackers, canned or packaged soups, processed cheeses, commercial salad dressings.

Calcium: *0-2 serving/week*

Kelp, cheese, turnip greens, brewer's yeast, parsley, corn tortillas, dandelion greens, Brazil nuts, watercress, milk, figs, yogurt, whole wheat, broccoli, cottage cheese, spinach, pecans, dried apricots.

Nitrogen (beef): *0-2 times/month*

Beef, red meats

Eat
Deficient Foods

Carbon: *1-2 servings/day*

Carbohydrates, starches, grains, breads, sweet fruits, oils [Eat foods without white sugar and corn syrup!]

Phosphorus: *1-2 servings/day*

Beans, black-eyed peas, butternuts, caviar, poultry (limited), seeds (pumpkin, squash, sunflower, sesame), gelatin, lentils, almonds, pinto beans, peanuts, walnuts, cashews, rye, scallops, oats, crab.

Sodium, Magnesium:
1-2 servings/day

Cashews, blackstrap molasses, buckwheat, dulse, millet, filberts, peanuts, walnuts, rye, coconuts, soybeans, strawberries, okra, sprouts, pineapples, cod, lamb, poultry, sesame seeds, carrots, nuts (not Brazil or pecan), collard leaves, sweet corn.

Eat...

Nitrogen (vegetable):
1-2 servings/day

Legumes (peas, beans), black-eyed peas, seeds, nuts (not Brazil and pecan), pasta, spirulina, soybean — as desired
Eggs, poultry, fish — 3-4 times weekly
Note: Eat any healthy foods you desire, but be sure to include type foods in your daily choices.

If Vegetarian:

If vegetarian, or needing more weight, take two tablespoons of protein powder in juice daily. Drink slowly to facilitate digestion. In this way, you may gain needed weight.

▶ *Approximate your food ratios. On any particular day, it does not matter if one meal is mostly alkaline and another mostly acid—just try to balance it out for the day! If you make a mistake, try again tomorrow. It is a subjective call that you make, as what you do over weeks and months makes the difference to your health.*

Note -

The food recommendations are for the generic type. Additionally, you may need from a holistic healer or nutritionist something more specific for your individuality.

―――――

Marasmic Nutritional Supplements

[Take all supplements with food.]

- **Multi-Vitamins** —
  1 capsule/day

- **Magnesium** —
  200 mg/day

- **Phosphorus** —
  2 tablets/day ('Phosfood' from Standard Process Lab.)

- **Do <u>not</u> take Calcium or Multi-Minerals** —
  You already have excessive calcium in your body. (Exception: if menopausal, on estrogen, or osteoporosis)

- **Herbs** —
  Brain detox – Chickweed or Valerian Rt.
  Organ detox – Fo-Ti or Elderberry Leaf
  (Take one capsule, twice daily for one month; then one, three times weekly.)
  Note: Be sure to take these supplements if you have ill-health. If in good health, take them at least 3-4 times/week.

Important Marasmic Health Concerns

You have weak vegetarian genetics and need the partial *vegetarian Food Guide*. You become over-acid and ill from eating excessive beef, chloride, and calcium foods.

After age 30-40, limit beef to 0-2 times monthly; other animal protein 3-4 days weekly is appropriate, with 2-3 vegetarian days weekly.

MARASMIC FOOD GUIDE

Aim for –
60% Fruits, salads, vegetables
40% Proteins, carbohydrates
and
50% Raw food diet
50% Cooked foods
Lose the saltshaker!
Be sure to take the recommended supplements.

Marasmic Weight Loss

Usually, for your health and healing, you need to gain some fat by increasing your daily calorie intake. But if holding excessive fat, then follow these instructions:

- *Gluten* sensitivity is common
- *Protein* drink daily, have about 25-30 grams
- *Eat* your body type deficient mineral foods daily
- *Follow* your *Marasmic Guide (as above)*
- *Exercise*: your body type requires only light daily exercise (like yoga, walking, roller-skating, etc.)
- *Simple sugars*: stop all white table sugar and high-fructose corn syrup and drinks containing these sugars
- *Mental balance and positive thinking:* you are very easily mentally stressed by everyday life, which causes adrenal hypoglycemia, low blood sugar; you need to take these supplements: *calcium/magnesium*, two capsules, twice daily with food; and *chamomile,* two capsules with food
- *Hypoglycemia:* this hormonal imbalance stops fat loss, and usually initiates more fat production, so it is vital to deal with this problem: take *pantothenic acid,* 500

mg/twice daily with food (see my earlier books to resolve this problem)

- *Calories:* As with any dietary approach, calories in must be *less than* calories out! Most markets sell a calorie booklet; make notes of your daily intake, and in most instances keep it under about 1500 calories/day

———

Thin Types
General Food Guide
(Vegetarian or Semi-Vegetarian)

Important Note

―――――

The Food Guide addresses the <u>Acid-Alkaline</u> aspect of your food intake, along with the <u>Type Mineral</u> factor presented throughout this book. It does <u>not</u> necessarily address calories or other dietary factors that may be pertinent to your personal health needs whether medical or appropriate for some other dietary need. So use your common sense and just include the factors described here with whatever healthy dietary choices you usually make.

For other nutrient information, consult with nutritional books or with holistic nutritional doctors. I particularly recommend the advice of Andrew Weil, M.D.

―――――

General Food Guide

This chapter presents a general Food Guide, upon which you superimpose the nutritional information from your type chapter.

————

Meat/Flesh Intake

Most muscle types should limit red meat to once or less weekly, while eggs, lamb, fish, or poultry are excellent in moderation. If ill or diseased, be sure to eat daily, one or two servings from each *deficient minerals* list. If not ill, eat them at least three times weekly for health maintenance. If this diet is similar to your present diet, but healing is sluggish, then:

- Decrease your carbohydrate and protein intake by about one-third
- Increase your fruit, salad, and vegetable intake by about one-third
- Consult with a holistic doctor, preferably one versed in nutritional and emotional evaluation

————

Over-Acid or Over-Alkaline?

Just as a log of wood burned in your fireplace leaves a mineral-ash, food ash refers to the minerals remaining after metabolizing foods in your tissues:

- Fruits, vegetables **alkalinize** tissues
- Proteins, carbohydrates **acidify** tissues

Usually You Are Over-Acid Due To:

- Excessive intake of dairy foods
- Excessive intake of proteins and carbohydrates
- Deficient intake of fruits, salads and vegetables
- Accumulated metabolic waste-acids (from years of eating excessive acid-ash foods, meats and carbohydrates, and from lack of exercise)
- You need to estimate the ratio of foods eaten. Generally, eat the following *approximate* ratios for your health:

60% <u>Alkaline-ash</u> foods *(fruits, salads, vegetables)*

40% <u>Acid-ash</u> foods *(complex carbohydrates like starches, grains, cereals, breads, flour products; and proteins)*

Approximate your food ratios. On any particular day, it does not matter if one meal is mostly alkaline, and another mostly acid—just try to balance it out for the day! If you get it wrong, try again tomorrow. It is a subjective call that you make, and it is what you do over weeks, months, or years that make the difference—not on any one or two days.

———

Important

- Minimize white sugar and alcohol intake.
- If desired, interchange lunches for dinners.
- Never eat foods you are allergic to, no matter what I recommend; if allergic, or suspect a food allergy, eliminate it and substitute from your type mineral lists.
- Eat the right foods 80-90% of the time and the Food Guide will work for you; unlike some types you do not have to live out of a health food store (although such foods are healthier for you).

▶ *Omit eating the excessive minerals in your type chapter, and be sure to eat one or two servings from the deficient list daily.*

On any particular day, it does not matter if one meal is mostly alkaline, and another mostly acid—just try to balance it out for the day! If you make a mistake, try again tomorrow. It is a subjective call that you make, and it is what you do over weeks, months, or years that make the difference—not on any one or two days or vweeks.

———

Acid/Alkaline Genetics, Dietary-Ash, and Raw Food Needs

This chart shows the Rocine types, their acid or alkaline food needs, and the percentage of raw foods needed for your health and healing.

- Apply your Type Minerals to the Food Guide

Type Genetics	Acid/Alkaline Genetics	% Food-Ash Needed	% Raw Food
Atrophic	*Acid*	*80% alkaline*	*90*
Exesthesic	*Acid*	*70% alkaline*	*70*
Marasmic	*Acid*	*60% alkaline*	*50*
Neurogenic	*Acid*	*70% alkaline*	*50*
Pathoferic	*Alkaline*	*50% alkaline*	*30*
Sillevitic	*Alkaline*	*50% alkaline*	*30*

The above percentages vary depending on aging and the health of individual types.

▶ *Observe the excessive minerals in your type chapter, and be sure to eat one or two servings from the deficient list daily (or, several times weekly).*

Important

- Minimize white sugar and alcohol intake.
- If desired, interchange lunches for dinners.
- Never eat foods you are allergic to no matter what is recommended; if allergic or suspect a food allergy, eliminate it and substitute from your type mineral lists.
- Eat the right foods 80-90% of the time and the *Food Guide* will work for you.
- You may have allergies to wheat, corn, other grains, sugar, alcohol, and milk (examine your body reactions to these foods for fatigue, sinusitis, joint pain, skin rash, and gastro-intestinal reactions). Note that the *atrophic* type *requires* dairy foods for health and healing.
- Living out of a health food store is unnecessary (although such foods are healthier for you). If you want dietary perfection in your healing efforts, eat organic foods (from a health food store).

In addition to your body type needs other holistic healing matters also need your attention. I suggest that you refer to my web site and earlier books for that information: *DrStenbeck.net*

———

Finally, in addition to your body type needs, other holistic healing matters also need your attention. I strongly suggest that you refer to my web site and earlier books for that information: *DrStenbeck.net*

———

General Food Guide

[Superimpose the nutritional information from your Type Chapter into this Food Guide.]

Breakfast

FRUIT *salad, fresh (with citrus fruit) and* <u>*protein:*</u> *yogurt, kefir, milk, cheeses, or raw seeds or nuts — 3+ times/week; or*

CEREALS *(whole grain), fruit, seeds, and nuts as desired — 2+ times/week; or*

EGGS *(1-2) with lettuce, tomato, veges, non-wheat toast — 0-3 times/week; or*

OTHER *choices — 0-1 times/week*

<u>*Daily Liquids*</u>

Coffee, teas — 0-1 cups
Pure water, citrus, fruit, or vegetable juices, soups, other — as desired
Wheat is a common allergy: avoid white breads; eat sour dough, millet, or oat breads instead.
Note: For in-between snacks, have fruit or vegetables, with seeds or nuts.

General Food Guide
<u>Lunch</u>

SALADS, *mixed green, with <u>protein</u> (cheese, soy, seeds, egg, etc.) Dressing: virgin olive oil and vinegar, low-fat dressings — 3-5 times weekly; and/or*

VEGETABLES with salad (and a <u>protein</u>: yogurt, cottage cheese...) — 1-3 times/week; or

FRUIT salad (like breakfast)
    — 1-2 times/week; or

SANDWICH, whole grains, cheese and /or other non-flesh <u>protein</u>; small salad
    — 0-2 times/week; or

OTHER choices
    — 0-1 times/week

* Other oils less ideal; soybean oil is a common allergen; minimize commercial dressings.

General Food Guide
Dinner

VEGETARIAN meals: include legumes, tofu, cheese, cottage cheese, seeds, nuts, egg, etc. (and/or salad) — 2+ times/week; or

POULTRY/FISH (3-6 oz.), salad and/or vegetables — 0-2 times/week; or

WHOLE GRAIN PASTA, cooked (barley, rice, millet, etc.), and salad/or vegetables — 0-2 times/week; or

OTHER choices — 1-2 times weekly

DESSERTS: Fruits, fresh or low-sugar desserts — as desired

Note: Be sure to include one or more selections from your type food lists in your daily food intake.

Note. Substitute flesh proteins with seeds, nuts, legumes, and other vegetables if *vegetarian.* You are vulnerable to being protein deficient so be careful to eat sufficient proteins and/or include a daily protein drink!

Food Guide Notes

Steamed Vegetables — Minerals are lost in the boiling of vegetables, so steaming or wok cooking is best.

Food Combinations — Eating proteins at the same meal with starches often results in indigestion, gas or constipation (as does eating fruit and starch together). For those of you with weak digestive systems, watch how this or other inharmonious combinations may be affecting you.

Periodic Detox Dieting — If you over-indulge in acid-ash foods, you need occasional elimination diets for tissue waste-acid removal, supervised by a nutritional doctor.

Minimize —
- Plums, cranberries, and their juices
- Commercial, sugared, and fatty salad dressings
- Red meats, processed meats, wines, alcohol, and milk
- Coffee, white sugar, fructose, and chemical sugar substitutes
- Exposure to drugs, environmental chemicals, pesticides
- Avoid eating allergic foods

Healthy Weight — You have a good ability to lose and control weight by following the Food Guide instructions. If you gain weight, the most common reason is liver or kidney irritation due to food allergies or negative emotions—the key is to eat non-allergic foods. The *atrophic and marasmic* types usually need to gain weight. (Obviously, if you have a medical condition that contradicts this advice, do not change your diet!)

———

In Conclusion

It is difficult to discern some *Thin* types from *Muscle* types (like the lean and strong *calciferic, nervimotive, and medeic* types). Study them well and you will see the differences.

———

Appendix

Brief Extracts from
The 22 Unique Body Types

Appendix A

Types
(Brief extract)

Type comes from 'typus' meaning an image or impression, the study of types being called typology.

▶ *Rocine: "A combination of mental and structural features is consistently found in people of the same type."*

Rocine wrote that all types are a mixture of positive and negative qualities. He based his work on the biochemical individuality of our *mineral* absorption and utilization. Of course, all minerals are absorbed, but he postulated that different types of people *selectively* absorb certain minerals, to a greater or lesser extent, requiring specific mineral foods for their enhanced health and healing.

▶ *The type information cannot predict what or who you will become, or how successful or not, but your type is capable of bringing a creative excellence to whatever you do in life. If your type has negative qualities that you disagree with, remember that they are only tendencies and may or may not manifest in you.*

This book enlarges on Rocine's premise (early 1900's), integrated with the later research of Herbert Sheldon, M.D., Ph.D., at Harvard University (1930's), along with my fifty years of observations and experience with this subject.

Comparing your shared physical (and sometimes psychological) descriptions with the Celebrity Lists further assists the identification of your type. It is not that you will look exactly like, or be a twin to, any particular celebrity. Look closely at a celebrity's features: face, profile, height, weight, head, etc. If you know something about their talents, beliefs, success and failure spheres, health and weight challenges, attitudes and behaviors, etc., then you get clues as to what your type may be.

———

Understanding Types and Sub-Types

Each of us has a clearly discernible dominant type. Visualize the celebrity examples from movies, politics, sports, the arts and public life, and try to identify with their physical features. Look for similar features, remembering that you will not recognize all attributes in yourself. You are not looking for your twin!

The sub-type issue is the main reason people of the same major type can look so different. Remember that a type description does not characterize you exactly, but depicts your individual variant of a type.

▶ *The type questionnaire pinpoints the major features of that type: if the celebrity examples are unhelpful, you may be an unusual variant (in which case ignore the celebrity issue and give yourself 7 points on Question 1).*

———

Minerals

Minerals are essential life nutrients that accelerate enzyme and chemical reactions and provide a basis for your body typing. Although found in all tissues, different minerals tend to be concentrated in certain organs, their presence or absence contributing to the healing of such tissues; e.g., zinc accelerates prostate healing; calcium and manganese promote bone, joint and connective tissue healing.

Specific foods nurture each type, some people needing meats for their health others needing a vegetarian diet. A high potassium diet nurtures one person, while another needs high sulfur, calcium, zinc, or another mineral.

Mineral Digestion and Absorption

Compared to vitamins, minerals are *difficult* to digest, absorb, and utilize. In people with strong digestive systems, this aspect may not be important. The following factors should be in place for optimal mineral metabolism:

1. Stomach Hydrochloric Acid Production
2. Parathyroid Hormone Balance
3. Organ Toxic Metal and Chemical Removal
   [See details in The 22 Unique Body Types.]

———

Total Body Healing

Note that from a holistic healing perspective, in addition to minerals and type information, the following healing factors are necessary:

> *Nutrient Balance*
> *Mental Balance*
> *Emotional Balance*
> *Spiritual Balance*
> *Detoxifying Integrity*

The above factors are all important to your total healing especially if you are interested in self-healing (see my earlier books).

———

Appendix B

Researchers
(Brief extract)

The predominant workers in this area of human individuality from around 1880's to the 1960's are Herbert Sheldon, M.D., Ph.D., Roger Williams, Ph.D., and Victor Rocine, D.Sc.

Much information on Sheldon's research exists on-line and in medical psychology libraries; for interested readers there are other lines of research published in the last century. This present book is primarily about Rocine's body types.

Herbert Sheldon M.D., Ph.D.

In contrast to Rocine, Sheldon at Harvard University in the 1930's was trained in the scientific method and did painstaking research and publishing on human individuality. In comparing his findings with Rocine's work, a direct putative correlation is visible.

Roger J. Williams, Ph.D.

Another significant researcher in human individuality is the renowned scientist and biochemist, Roger J. Williams. He demonstrated that different people have varying levels of nutrients, enzymes, and other metabolic chemicals in their bloodstreams.

▶ *Williams's research firmly expands on the premise of individual nutritional needs in human beings. If interested in his research, I highly recommend his book Biochemial Individuality.*

Victor Rocine, D.Sc.

Note that when a negative feature is indicated, say neurotic tendencies, all members of the type are <u>not</u> that way; it is a type tendency reported by Rocine.

Rocine studied type-related diseases finding links between mineral and dietary factors with individual types and their diseases. In each body type, one or more dominant minerals are preferentially absorbed and utilized over other minerals.

He recognized discrete body types from their physical appearance finding genetically based mineral dominance to be the determining feature. He also correlated their physical features with psychological characteristics.

―――

Appendix C

Genetics, Types, and Diet
(Brief extract)

This section deals with how nervous system genetics helps determine your eating choices for health: you are either born to be a predominant meat eater, a partial or complete vegetarian, or something between the two. The genetic factor determining this dietary aspect is the *sympathetic and parasympathetic* components of your central nervous system. This represents a basic factor in eating for health.

This chapter helps you understand your dietary inheritance, although instinctively, you may already have arrived there!

- If born **sympathetic** dominant you are *genetically acid*, desiring a predominantly *vegetarian* diet for your health (about 70% fruit, salad, vegetables to 30% proteins and carbohydrates).

- If born **parasympathetic** dominant you are *genetically alkaline*, desiring a predominantly *carnivorous* diet for your health (about 70% proteins, carbohydrates to 30% fruits, salads, vegetables). Few of you ever choose to become vegetarian because of the difficulty in satisfying your protein needs without meats.

- If born *intermediate* dominant you may eat food groups with little concern for the acid/alkaline factor. However, after age 40, you need a semi-vegetarian diet for healthy eating.

———

Chart of Relative Nervous System Dominance

In the following Chart, if you relate to many of the symptoms on one side you probably have that nervous system dominance; relating to both sides indicates *Intermediate* dominance.

If Vegetarian (Over-acid) --
Eat 70% fruits, salads, vegetables
And 30% proteins, carbohydrates

If Carnivore (Over-alkaline) --
Eat 70% proteins, carbohydrates
And 30% fruits, salads, vegetables

If Intermediate --
Eat 50:50 of acid and alkaline-ash foods

Make an *approximate* estimate of your daily acid and alkaline food intake (such ratios varying from type to type).

———

Symptoms of Relative Genetic Dominance

Vegetarians (Over-acid)	*Carnivores* (Over-alkaline)
Sympathetic Dominance	*Parasympathetic Dominance*
little or no flesh desire	*desire flesh*
easily constipated	*rarely constipated*
slow digestion	*fast digestion*
easily dehydrated	*not dehydrated*
strong thirst	*low thirst*
pale face	*flushed face*
high pulse after food	*slow pulse after food*
easy gag reflex	*slow gag reflex*
cool dry skin	*moist warm skin*
nervous stomach	*calm stomach*
little eyelid blinking	*much blinking*
nervous tendency	*mostly calm*
slower healing	*faster healing*
low oxygen-uptake	*good oxygen-uptake*
easily breathless	*seldom breathless*
insomnia common	*sleep easier*
few muscle cramps	*some night cramps*
calcium deposits rare	*get calcium deposits*

Appendix D

Help Identifying your Body Type with Dr. Stenbeck

If you desire help in identifying your body type, follow these instructions, and answer the questionnaire. For further information and fees, send me an email from page one of the website:

DrStenbeck.net

First name: _____

Country of birth: _____

Upload photos and send to the above website:

- Head and shoulders: front and side views

- Full body: front and side views

- Also 1-2 teenage views

- If possible, casual photos of mother, father, siblings

MY TYPE CLASS MAY BE: _____

   (Thin, Muscle, or Fat)

AGE   -   _____

HEIGHT   -   _____ feet/inches

MY WEIGHT -   _____ pounds

   Heaviest at age: _____

- Lightest as adult: _____

- Estimate age 15: _____

VISION - Excellent Average   Poor:

HAIR -   Natural color: _____

- Thin/thick? _____

- balding? _____

SKIN - Quality: _____

- History of acne, boils, other:

_____

_____

TEETH   - Strong   Weak   Dentures

- Cavity history: Many   Moderate   Few

MUSCLES - Strong   Average   Weak

Sports played _____

JOINTS   - Strong   Average   Weak

HEALTH - Childhood diseases?

_____

_____

- Adult diseases?

_____

AVERAGE DIET

- Beef _____ (times/week)

- Poultry _____ (times/week)

- Fish _____ (times/week)

- Eggs _____ (times/week)

- Water _____ (glasses/day):

- Vegetarian? Vegan? _____

- Other? _____

- Did your childhood diet differ? _____

The above will help me know who you are! I will send you a follow-up questionnaire for further help in identifying your body type.

Appendix E

On-line Health Consultation with Dr. Stenbeck

For further information, or to comment on this book, or to receive a response on any health issue from a holistic viewpoint, send an email inquiry from page one of my website:

DrStenbeck.net

Following that, I will suggest further healing needs, which we may pursue with an on-line consult.

———

Appendix F

Notes

See my book <u>*The 22 Unique Body Types,*</u> available at the usual online source, for further information and details on all of the 22 Types. The Appendix in that book has further information about:

Mineral Functions and Food Sources

Further Reading

———

www.ingramcontent.com/pod-product-compliance
Lightning Source LLC
Chambersburg PA
CBHW071229280526
45787CB00002B/855